OLIVE FLAME WEIGHTLOSS DIET BOOKLET

For quick, easy, and affordable Fatloss, Fitness, & Fabulosity

by

Humphrey Zinyuke (R.Nutr)

Copyright

Book Title: Olive Flame Weightloss Diet Booklet
Book Author: Humphrey Zinyuke
© 2013, Humphrey Zinyuke
hzinyuke@yahoo.com

ISBN: 978-1-304-48503-8

"Beloved I wish above all things that you may prosper and be in good health even as your soul prospers..." - **3 John 1: 2**

Table of Contents

Welcome

Congratulations on taking practical steps to take control of your health and manage your weight. If weightloss is your ambition, whether for purposes of fatloss, fitness, or fabulosity then you are definitely on the right track. The Olive Flame Weightloss Program was designed and perfected by a qualified Nutritionist, who has acquired years of experience working in the medical field of Nutrition as well as Public Health Research. Having invested much time and effort studying both the perceived strengths/positives and the perceived weaknesses/negatives of some of the world's leading weightloss programs such as: the amazing The Dr. Cohen Diet, The Blood Type Diet, Atkins Diet, Weight Watchers, The Fatloss Lab, and The Mediterranean Diet, amongst others, the author harnessed this wealth of knowledge and decided to fulfill his calling to assist the millions out there struggling with weight management with this simple, affordable, and highly effective weightloss program. The only thing we at Olive Flame Nutrition Company ask of you from the onset is that you make a firm decision and pinpoint on a scale of 1 to 10 exactly how important your weightloss ambitions are to you. The more determined you are the easier it will be for you to sail through. Remember, nothing great has ever been done without enthusiasm. Once again, congratulations and all the best!

Overview

The Olive Flame Weightloss Program hinges on correct and consistent adherence to the structured day-by-day nutrition/eating plan. The program does not come with a detailed physical exercise plan, although even as shall be mentioned towards the end of this nutrition guide, physical exercise is always undoubtedly part and parcel of both healthy living and effective weight management and is thus generally recommended. Expert guidelines on physical exercise are provided at the end.

With the Olive Flame Weightloss Program you are presented with a scientifically sound nutrition program that gives you the opportunity to lose between 5-15kgs in a period of between 2-8weeks on average. It must be highlighted early on that the Olive Flame Weightloss Program is not another diet fad with a beginning and an end. It is, rather, an introduction to a model or template for a healthier nutritional approach that one can model their everyday eating patterns along for a lifetime so as to ensure lifelong healthy weight and vitality.

This Olive Flame Weightloss Diet Booklet is designed to assist its users by offering support in two areas that work hand-in hand, namely:

i. A personalized nutrition/eating plan, with the option of Blood Type based food choices. ii. As well as lifestyle and physical exercise advisory guidelines.

You will be pleased to learn that the Olive Flame Program is holistic in its approach in that it aims to address the 8-Pillars of an excellent weight management program (according to research on patient requirements), namely:

a. Strategically adjusting Patient Caloric (Energy) Intake to support fat-burning.
b. Balancing Carbohydrate-Protein-Fat intake proportions to ensure weightloss.
c. Empathizing with and working around the reality of patients' mood-based eating patterns.
d. Incorporating an all-important detoxification component into the fatloss program, with optional guidelines on Blood Type based food choices. e. Managing appetite and ensuring fullness/satiety.
f. Educating and advising patients on physical exercise best practices.

g. Catering for the all-important need for hormonal balance in fatloss.
h. Supporting optimal bowel movement, thus minimizing or preventing constipation.

Some Key Points

- The Olive Flame Weightloss Program is based on correct and consistent adherence to the structured day-to-day nutrition/eating plan as found in the diet booklet.

- The selection of food items and food groups/classes used during this program is guided by preference of low Glycemic Index (low G.I) food items, as well as overall low calorie (low-energy) intake that is crucial for the burning of undesirable, excess fat in your body.

- Because the burning of fat generally produces more energy than alternative energy sources, after 4 days of starting the program, at which stage the fatburning process is typically 'triggered', patients will generally start to feel more energetic and less hungry. It must be noted that the Olive Flame Weight Loss Program targets merely the undesirable, excess fat deposits in the body; such as the thigh area, the arms, the belly etc.

- If the program is followed correctly, one can expect safe and exciting weight-loss of 5-15kgs in 2-8weeks on average. However, this is STRICTLY ON CONDITION THAT THE EATING PLAN IS FOLLOWED RELIGIOUSLY.

Ideally the maximum total calorie (energy) intake per day during this program will and should average no more than 1200 calories/day. Any failure to lose weight steadily (i.e. 0.4kg -0.6kg per day) means that one is 'cheating', particularly on the calorie intake limit. As such one must experiment and cut down certain food portions to revamp the fat-burning process anytime weightloss slows down or stalls.

- The Olive Flame Weightloss Program recommends and facilitates an average daily calorie intake of 1000calories per day. Many scientists agree that this figure is practical, in comparison with many of the highly calorie-restrictive, hormone, homogenous-hormone, or placebo-based diet programs marketed on the internet. Many of these diets restrict daily caloric intake to 500calories, a level which many medical scientists argue does support weightloss but is too restrictive to be practical for the average person's day to day routine.

- The Olive Flame Weightloss Program also accommodates Vegetarians, thus alternative foods for different kinds of vegetarians are also mentioned in the program.

- The Olive Flame Program is structured in the form of Four (4) phases, whose names and nature shall be mentioned in this booklet.

- The Olive Flame Program comes with optional Blood Type based eating guidelines. Dieters who, based on authentic medical records, are aware of their blood type have the option of refining their weightloss program as guided by the Blood Type Dietary Guidelines section toward the very end of this manual.

Although generally recommended, the idea of making food choices based on one's blood type is entirely optional and individuals on the Olive Flame program CAN ignore that section, be it because they do not have the means to have their Blood Type professionally verified, or they simply do not subscribe to the concept of Blood Type based eating. The Blood Type Dietary Guidelines Tables are courtesy of Michael Lam, MD, MPH, of the *Blood Type Diet* fame. (www.DrLam.com)

A Few Ground Rules

- DO NOT follow the Olive Flame Weightloss Program if: you are certain or suspect that you may be pregnant, if you are exclusively breastfeeding, if you have been medically diagnosed of kidney (renal) disease or failure, or if you are using Diuretic drugs.

- Please note that Doctors warn about serious health problems caused by mixing certain medicines and Grapefruit. There are currently some 85 such drugs, including statins, antibiotics, antidepressants, drugs to treat cancer and heart disease, plus others used by patients who have had organ transplants. According to a report in the Canadian Medical Association Journal, Grapefruit contains a compound, furanocoumarin, that prevents enzymes in the intestine, responsible for keeping foreign substances out of the body, from working properly. Grapefruit can either increase the potency of drugs, potentially leading to an overdose, or render them less effective which puts patients at risk of receiving too little medication.

- Please use the Body Mass Index (BMI) system to get an idea of whether or not you are medically classified as obese, overweight, under-weight or of healthy weight. See how to calculate BMI at the end of this manual.

- Be sure to emulate the free online template(s) provided to draft and keep a food diary, ensuring that you capture accurately your daily food intake for monitoring purposes. This food diary will help you make the necessary adjustments in the event that your weightloss stalls and you need to cut down on your food portions. Once again, please imitate the free illustrative food diary outlines provided, or design one on a computer and print or photocopy as many sheets as you may need for the duration of your program. In addition, please ensure you drink a minimum of 2litres of water per day.

- If for some reason you falter or deviate from the diet and eat more at any stage before the Stabilization Phase, DO NOT quit nor go on a guilt trip. Remind yourself that nobody is perfect, and that if so many others have lost weight on the Olive Flame Program before then SO CAN YOU. Pick yourself up, recommit yourself to discipline and just keep going. You will make it. - If struggling with an addiction to certain food item(s), begin to cut them down gradually rather than to be discouraged and quit. Habits often take time to break.

- Sweets and chewing gum are not allowed during the program (with the exception of sugar-free gum).

- Aim to consume an average of 2 cloves of Garlic each day, whether eaten raw or used in cooking. Some helpful spices include Ginger, Cinnamon, Cayenne Pepper, Mustard Seed, & Black Pepper.

- Alcohol is high in calories (energy) and is best avoided or taken as moderately as possible. Alcohol also reduces self-control, making it harder to maintain the discipline necessary for the program. Not all alcohol is entirely harmful though. Red Wine in particular contains a good antioxidant Resveratrol, which can help prevent blockage of blood vessels, infertility, inflammation, and cardiovascular (heart) disease. As such, daily alcohol intake guidelines (if alcohol is to be taken at all) are as follows: 150ml (5 fl ounces) of wine, 350ml (12 fl ounces) of beer, or 45ml (1.5 ounces) of spirits.

- Many Cosmetics such as body lotions contain 'fats' which the body absorbs through the skin. These absorbed 'fats' then go on to contribute to a person's total daily fat or calorie intake, in addition to dietary intake. This additional fat can significantly slow down or stop weightloss. As such, for a limited period of about 6 weeks or even for the entire duration of your weightloss program, avoid using any cosmetic products that contain oils, fats, gels or vitamins. Instead, rather opt for only natural make-ups and care products. Baby oil and/ or natural mineral oil are best for dry-skinned people.

- One of the greatest hindrances to weightloss even when one is following a weightlloss eating program is consistently high levels of the hormone Cortisol in the blood. Cortisol (also known as the stress hormone) is good in preparing for emergency reactions (fight or flight). However when it is over-produced by the body it often promotes the deposition of fat around the abdominal area, as well as slowing down the functioning of the Thyroid Gland, thereby promoting weight gain. Some of the best ways to curb this problem is to manage stress and to cut down on or avoid consuming Caffeine (found in Caffeinated Coffee).

- The Blood Type based dietary guidelines toward the end of the manual, although recommended, are NOT compulsory and dieters can simply follow the general 4 Phase program without Blood Type consideration if they so wish.

Overall Eating Plan Outline

The Olive Flame Weightloss Program is structured into 4 phases as explained below:

⁵ʰₐₐₑᵗ ₑᵐ ₑ	⁴ᵗˣ ᴸₐˣⁱ́ᴘᵐ	⁵ᵗˣ ᴸᴬᴬₐₑ
⁵ʰₐₐₑ⁻ -"◆ᵐᵐ⁻ₓ ₐ́ ⁵ʰₐₐₑ"	◄ᵈʜₐ²ᵈ	This is a fat-loading phase where you feast on tasty fat-rich and carbohydrate-rich foods that you like. It is a prerequisite for a sustained low-calorie eating program. It triggers your fat-burning center in the brain to prepare for fat-burning, as well as stocking up your essential fat-cells. This stage is scientifically proven to be extremely important and not to be skipped.
⁵ʰₐₐₑ◄ₐ_"⁺ ₐkₑᴹff ⁵ʰₐₐₑ"	◄⁻ʜₐ²ᵈ	This phase marks the beginning of the exciting Fat-burning process. After about 5days on this phase, dieters will begin to notice changes. For some, the duration of the "Take Off Phase" will be enough for them to lose all the weight they wish to lose, before proceeding straight to the "Touch-down/Stabilization Phase". It is quite possible to lose anything between 5-15kgs in these 21days. This phase MUST be completed by anybody on the program regardless of how little the desired weightloss may be.
⁵ʰₐₐₑ◄ₐ_ᵗᵗ ᵐᵐᵈₑ⁻ ᴴᴴₑ ⁵ʰₐₐₑ"	ᴹₐᴸⁱᴘᵐ ₐ|ᵐᵐ ᴴₑᴸ ʜfᵛᴹ_ʜₐᵛ ⁊⁊◄ꟾₑₐ. ⁵ᴸᴘˣ ᴹꟾ◄⁊ꟾₑₐ ◄ᴴ ₐₑᵛ ₑ⁻ₐꟾᵐ ᴘᴹᵗʰₐ ᵐᵐ ₐᴴₑᵗᴴ Ħf ⁊⁊ᴘᵐ ₐₑᴘˣᴸᵛ ₑᵛᴹ_ ʜₐᵛ ⁊⁊ꟾₑₐ	The "Cruise Mode Phase" is for those who, after the 21-day "Take Off Phase" feel they still have more weight to lose. It gives the dieter room for sustained-weightloss. During this phase dieters who have set a target weight for themselves have the option of going on an unlimited number of 10day cycles, ranging from 1 (one) 10-day cycle to several months made up of consecutive 10-day cycles until they approximate their target weight.
⁵ʰₐₐₑ ℱ_ᵗᵗ ᴘᴴᶠʰ ◄ꟾ◄ᵐᵐ₇ₐᵗₐₚꟾᵗₐˣⁱᴘᵐ ⁵ʰₐₐₑ"	◄⁻ʜₐᵛ ᵈ	This is the stabilization phase of the program, whereby your body is being taught to get used to your new weight. It involves you eating larger portions of food from a wider variety of healthy foods. Your total caloric intake will also have gone up.

Phase 1: "Runway Phase" (DAY 1 & DAY 2)

FAT FEAST

Although this often contradicts many people's traditional beliefs about fat, on the first 2days go ahead and feast on high-fat and high carbohydrate containing foods that you enjoy. If you are Diabetic, control the sugar/carbohydrate intake as usual but do gorge yourself on tasty high-fat foods especially.

Examples of foods to be taken include Dairy products such as Yoghurt, Butter, and Cheeses, as well as Eggs, Oils, Seeds, Avocadoes, Olives, Peanut Butter, different kinds of Nuts, Mayonnaise, Whipped Cream etc.

Phase 2: "Take-Off Phase" (DAY 3 - DAY 23)

1000 Calorie, Low Carbohydrate Diet.

Starting from the 3rd day begin to follow the 1000calorie per day, low carbohydrate eating guidelines described below as religiously as possible. A typical day will include 3 meals and 2 snacks-in between the 3 main meals. Do not worry about counting-calories. The program is designed to predetermine that for you.

With regards to food preparation you are encouraged to use healthy cooking methods such as boiling, steaming, baking, grilling or "braaing" as much as possible. However, if anything is to be fried at all then use an extremely minimal amount of Olive oil (especially), or Canola oil, Safflower oil, Sunflower oil, or other Vegetable oils. It must be emphasized that the best oil to use is Extra Vegan Olive Oil that is carried in dark (opaque) containers which do not permit light to reach the oil. This protection prevents the oil from becoming rancid, thereby losing its numerous, all-important health benefits.

Breakfast

Regardless of what combination of food items you will choose from the different breakfasts suggested below, the bottom line is that you must aim to have at least 20-30grams of Protein early in the morning for breakfast. Good protein sources for breakfast include: Egg white, 1 hard-boiled whole egg, 1 scrambled egg, omelet, 1/2-1 whole sausage, Cottage Cheese (or other cheeses especially 'White Cheeses'), Greek Yoghurt, Skim Milk, Soy Milk, Salmon (Fish), Bacon, or a good Protein Shake. Choose any 1 of these or a sensible combination as a 'Protein Source' in the morning.

EITHER

i] 2 Weetbix strips in 150ml of Skimmed Milk/Soy Milk (artificially sweetened i.e. no
Table Sugar) or in 150ml or less of 100% Fruit Juice + any 1 of the following
Fruits: 1 Apple, 1/2 Grapefruit, 6-8 Strawberries, 6-8 Plums, 1 Peach, 1-2

Naartjies, Watermelon, 1/3 Paw Paw, or 1/2 an English Cucumber. (The dieter has the option of omitting the fruit)

OR

ii] Any number of cups of Decaffeinated Coffee, Tea, or Herbal Tea (especially
Green Tea) - artificially sweetened + 1 Slice Wholegrain Bread with a Protein source such as Peanut Butter. [The dieter is best advised to avoid sugar and to rather use Lemon (juice) or 1 Stevia sweetener if they have a sweet-tooth. 1 or 2 teaspoons of sugar are only advisable if feeling dizzy or experiencing headaches.]

Snack

Any 1 of the following: 1/2 a Cucumber, 1/2 Apple, 1/2 Grapefruit, 1/2 Orange,
80ml Fat-free/Plain/Natural Yoghurt, a reasonable amount of Provita Biscuits (5 or less), Cracker Bread, or Rice Cakes, or a maximum of 1 Liter of Sprite Zero or Tab (No Coke Zero or Fanta Zero).

This snack is entirely optional. For purposes of rapid weightloss, the dieter that does not have the snack is at an advantage over the dieter that does have one, although the snack helps stabilize blood sugar resulting in curbed feelings of hunger and overeating.

Lunch

Lunch will be made up from a combination of PROTEIN, together with either VEGETABLES or a MIXED SALAD. A cup of Green Tea (without sugar but with an optional Stevia Sweetener or Lemon (juice) if preferred) is also advisable.

PROTEIN: 100g (measured raw) of any 1 of these meats: Lean Beef (no visible fat), Skinless Chicken (especially chicken breast), Tuna/Canned Fish (in brine,
i.e. salt-solution only), Fish (especially but not exclusively Talapia, Salmon, Sardines, Mackerel, Halibut, Herring, Bream, Sole, Plaice), or Turkey. As an alternative to these meats you can have any one of these: 85g Cottage Cheese

(OR any other White Cheeses such as Greek or Italian Mozzarella Cheese), 1 Boiled Egg, 4 Egg Whites, 150g Tofu, or 180ml Plain/Natural Yoghurt.

(Vegetarians can rather use 75-100g Tofu, 100g Vegetarian Sausages, 150-200g Soy Yoghurt, 85g Cottage Cheese, 3 Egg Whites, or 180ml Plain/Natural Yoghurt, or simply enjoy the variety of vegetables) Together with EITHER:

i] VEGETABLES: An unlimited but sensible amount of a combination of any of the following vegetables: Cabbage, Cauliflower, Broccoli, Asparagus, Peppers (green, orange, red, yellow), Celery, Spinach, Green Beans, Onions, Garlic, Radishes, Cucumber, Tomatoes, Okra, Mushrooms, Kale, Leeks, Chard, Chicory or other Green Leafy Vegetables.

OR

ii] SALAD: An unlimited but sensible amount of Vegetable Salad, comprising any combination of: lettuce, greens such as cabbage, cucumber, onion, and tomato. A simple salad dressing would constitute a few teaspoons of Olive Oil and/or Lemon Juice. Another idea for Salad Dressing is Apple Cider Vinegar, Balsamic Vinegar, or any sugar-free Vinegar of choice. No fatty or sugary salad creams or mayonnaise.

Snack

Any 1 of the following: 1/2 a Cucumber, 1/2 Apple, 1/2 Grapefruit, 1/2 Orange, 80ml Fat-free/Plain/Natural Yoghurt, a reasonable amount of Provita Biscuits (5 or less), Cracker Bread, or Rice Cakes, or a maximum of 1 Liter of Sprite Zero or Tab (No Coke Zero or Fanta Zero).
This snack is entirely optional. For purposes of rapid weightloss, the dieter that does not have the snack is at an advantage over the dieter that does have one, al-
though the snack helps stabilize blood sugar resulting in curbed feelings of hunger and overeating.

Dinner

Dinner under the Olive Flame Weightloss Program can be worked out using the same choices as those that apply to Lunch. For purposes of variety, you are advised to avoid repeating the same choices of meat and/or vegetables as those you would have had for lunch in the same day. Variety has been said to be the essence of life. So for instance, if you had a particular combination of vegetables for lunch, you may want to then enjoy a salad in the evening instead, and vice-versa! A cup of Green Tea [without sugar but with an optional Stevia Sweetener or Lemon (juice) if preferred] is also advisable.

NB: *The dieter is allowed to rearrange their daily food portions whichever way they may like throughout the day, as long as they do not exceed the daily portion limits. It is however important to avoid taking high-calorie foods all at the same time, such as two fruits within 2 hours of each other.*

Phase 3: "Cruise Mode Phase" (Day 24 onwards)

1000 Calorie, Low Carbohydrate Diet.

The "Cruise Mode Phase" is for those who, after the preceding 21-day "Take Off Phase" feel they still have more weight to lose. It gives the dieter room for steady, sustained-weightloss. During this phase dieters who have set a target weight for themselves have the option of going on an unlimited number of consecutive 10day cycles, ranging from 1 (one) 10-day cycle to several months made up of consecutive 10-day cycles until they approximate their target weight.

The "Cruise Mode Phase" is optional and those dieters who after the preceding 21day Take Off Phase feel they have lost all or most of the weight they wanted to lose rapidly can now freely proceed to the next and final phase of the program as described below.

On the other hand, if after the preceding 21-day "Take Off Phase" you feel you still have a considerable amount of weight to lose you can now simply continue to follow the guidelines of the "Take-Off Phase" in their exact form strictly, 10 days at a time. Depending on how many kilos you wish to still lose, the number of your 10day cycles can range from just 1(one) to several months made up of consecutive 10-day cycles [8-11 month long success stories are possible and marvelous].

If at any given point during this phase you feel that your target weight is afar off and you now need to take a break, you can proceed to do your 14day Stabilization/"Touch Down" Phase, take a break, and simply start the program all over again in its strict form from the top when ready. During your break you will have increased your portions of healthy foods, and possibly include controlled portions of unrefined carbohydrate.

Phase 4: "Touch Down/Stabilization Phase"

1000+ Calorie, Low Carbohydrate Diet.

The Stabilization or "Touch Down" phase of the program is a phase whereby your body is now being taught to get used to your new weight. It involves you eating larger portions of food from a wider variety of healthy foods. Your total caloric intake will also understandably have gone up.

The stabilization phase must of necessity last for 21days, which is the approximate time it takes for your body to maintain your new-found weight. During this phase you are allowed to increase the portion sizes of the foods you have been taking all along, including Protein (meat), and Vegetables. Previously disallowed fruits that are high on the Glycemic Index (G.I) such as Bananas, Pineapple, and Mangoes are now permissible in moderation. You are, however, still keeping your carbohydrate intake at the same minimal levels as in preceding phases, including avoiding Carbohydrates after 4.00pm (i.e. 1600hrs).

Below is an example of a "Stabilization Phase" Meal Plan for a day:

Breakfast

Decaffeinated Coffee/ Green Tea + 2 Eggs (boiled or omelet)/2 Slices Ham/Bacon + 1 Slice Whole Wheat Toast+ 25g Avocado + 1Raw Tomato.

OR

High Fibre Cereal (especially Oatmeal) in 150ml of Low Fat Milk (no sugar) + any 1 of the following Fruits: 1 Apple, 1/2 Grapefruit, 8 Strawberries, 8 Plums,
1 Peach, 1 Naartjie, Watermelon, 1/3 Paw Paw, or 1/2 an English Cucumber, Mango, Pineapple.

Snack

EITHER
Any 1 of the following: 1/2 a Cucumber, 1/2 Apple, 1/2 Grapefruit, 1/2 Orange, 8 Strawberries, 100g Fat-free/Plain/Natural Yoghurt, a reasonable amount of Provita Biscuits (5 or less), Cracker Bread, or Rice Cakes, or a maximum of 1 Liter per day of Sprite Zero or Tab (No Coke Zero or Fanta

Zero). This snack is entirely optional. For purposes of rapid weightloss, the dieter that does not have the snack is at an advantage over the dieter that does have one, although the snack helps stabilize blood sugar resulting in curbed feelings of hunger and overeating.

OR

Any other of the sweeter fruits in season, e.g.:8 Plums, 1 Peach, 1-2 Naartjies, Watermelon, 1/3 Paw Paw, or 1 Mango, or 1/2 Pineapple.

Lunch

Grilled/ Fried Fish + 1/2-1 cup mixed salad in low fat dressing + 1 cup herbal Tea [without sugar but with an optional Stevia Sweetener or Lemon (juice) if preferred]

Snack

EITHER

Any 1 of the following: 1/2 a Cucumber, 1/2 Apple, 1/2 Grapefruit, 1/2 Orange, 8 Strawberries, 100g Fat-free/Plain/Natural Yoghurt, a reasonable amount of Provita Biscuits (5 or less), Cracker Bread, or Rice Cakes, or a maximum of 1 Liter per day of Sprite Zero or Tab (No Coke Zero or Tab). This snack is entirely optional. For purposes of rapid weightloss, the dieter that does not have the snack is at an advantage over the dieter that does have one, although the snack helps stabilize blood sugar resulting in curbed feelings of hunger and overeating.

OR

Any other of the sweeter fruits in season, e.g.:8 Plums, 1 Peach, 1-2 Naartjies, Watermelon, 1/3 Paw Paw, or 1 Mango, or 1/2 Pineapple.

Dinner

Grilled/Fried Chicken Breast (or Drumsticks) + Steamed Vegetables + 1 cup Green Tea [without sugar but with an optional Stevia Sweetener or Lemon (Juice) if preferred]

Beyond the "Touch Down/Stabilization Phase"

Seeing that you have attained your target weight, or at least stabilized your new-weight which is much better than where you used to be, what next? Well first of all congratulate yourself for a fight well fought. You have reason to be proud.

Secondly, ask yourself, in consultation with your Body Mass Index, as well as Doctor or Nutritionist if there is still need for you to lose more weight. If need be then you may start the program all over again. If, on the other hand, you are content with your new weight, you may now begin your new life with your new weight. Go ahead and begin also to gradually bring back into your diet healthy, unrefined, high-fiber carbohydrates that will not jeopardize your new weight, such as: Whole-grain bread, Oatmeal, High-Fiber Cereals (such as All Bran, Low -sugar muesli etc), Brown Rice etc. Similar to followers of the healthy Mediterranean Diet, it is at this juncture wise to aim at consuming an average of 1-4 cups of beans (different kinds) everyday as a healthy source of carbohydrate. Include things such as Chickpeas, Black Beans, and Lentils.

Tips, Tit-Bits, and Trouble Shooting

- The term Body Mass Index (B.M.I) refers to a scientific measure of how proportionate an individual's weight is to their height, from a health perspective. It is used to gauge whether one can be classified as being underweight, of normal weight, overweight, or obese.

Body Mass Index

Interpreting B.M.I
The term Body Mass Index (B.M.I) refers to a scientific measure of how proportionate an individual's weight is to their height, from a health perspective. It is used to gauge whether one can be classified as being underweight, of normal weight, overweight, or obese.

$$\text{Body Mass Index (B.M.I)} = \frac{\text{weight (in kgs)}}{\text{height}^2 \text{ (in meters)}} = \frac{\text{weight (in kgs)}}{\text{height} \times \text{height(m)}} \quad \text{e.g.} \quad \frac{86}{1.64 \times 1.64} = 32$$

I. B.M.I < 20 is classified as being underweight.

II. $20 \leq$ B.M.I ≤ 25 is classified as being in the normal/ideal weight range.

III. $25 \leq$ B.M.I ≤ 30 is classified as being overweight, but not obese.

IV. B.M.I > 30 is classified as being obese.

V. B.M.I > 40 is classified as extreme/ morbid obesity.

- It is normal for some people to experience headaches during the program. This can simply be solved by taking an over-the-counter pain-killer like Aspirin. Also remember to take the 2litres of water per day as mentioned earlier. Water can be still, borehole, carbonated, or any kind of clean water.

- Sticking to your weightloss program whilst needing to attend events such as parties, family gatherings and other social events can be quite a challenge. The way to handle this is to predetermine beforehand that you will stick to lean meats and vegetables. Avoid sugary condiments, such as Sauces and Fruit Chutneys. Also discipline yourself to try and avoid alcohol or stick to the stipulated ratio

- A plateau is any season/period during your weightloss program when the scale seems stuck and you seem to have stopped losing weight. Plateaus are common, normal, and no basis for one to panic or lose heart. They are caused by a number of different things. The following are some tips on how to overcome a plateau.

a. Remain resolute. Don't panic or be discouraged. In fact, it is both wise and advisable for you to ask supportive family and friends around you to support you whilst you are on the program. Please also make the effort to find at least one other supportive person who is either also can work together and support each other daily. THIS IS OF PARAMOUNT IMPORTANCE

b. Review your Food Diary to check compliance with the recommended food intake levels (portions), or if you have been taking forbidden food items.

c. Try cutting down food portions, especially by halving fruit portions, grilling rather than frying foods, and cutting down on starchy vegetables. Also cut out alcohol. Alcohol causes dehydration, leading to water retention. Also cut down on salt, as Sodium also promotes water   retention.

d. Check your water intake. If not satisfactory then increase it.

e. Try to increase your level of physical activity. Mild or moderate exercise should suffice.

f. Do a Turbo Boost Day. On this day take no food both in the morning and afternoon, except for either water, tea, or coffee with no sugar. For dinner, proceed to then take your typical serving of protein (meat product) plus a fruit of choice, like an apple or 6-8 strawberries. *Remember to take a total of at least 2 Liters of water throughout the day.*

- Be sure you get sufficient sleep. Lack of sleep and/or relaxation can promote weight gain. This is also closely linked to Stress which results in overproduction of the stress hormone Cortisol. Cortisol promotes the deposition of fat especially around the abdominal area, whilst also affecting the regulation of blood sugar levels- which then leads to increased appetite for starchy, fatty and sugary foods.

- Individuals with suspected or confirmed Thyroid problems must seek medical attention as suppressed Thyroid function often implies weight gain.
- The usage of certain Nutritional Supplements is advisable during the Olive Flame Weightloss program. It is advisable for the dieter to get two sets of nutritional supplements. One must be a Multivitamin/Multinutrient Supplement that contains the full spectrum of micronutrients. The second nutritional supplement we strongly recommend is one specifically containing the Essential Fatty Acids known as Omega 3 Fatty Acids ONLY. It is advisable to take this supplement by itself, separate from the time you take the

Multivitamin supplement as some micronutrients in the multivitamin supplement can impede the optimal absorption of the Omega 3 Fatty Acids in the intestines.

Some of your daily nutrient requirements are covered by the program as shown:

Magnesium: Meat Products.
Copper: Meats and Fish.
Phosphorous: Beef, Chicken, Turkey, and Fish.
Potassium: Vegetables and Fruits.
Selenium: Wholegrains, Eggs, Fish.
Zinc: Fish, Beef, Whole grains, Vegetables.
Calcium: Fish, Vegetables, Fish, Dairy Products.
Iron: Beef, Green Leafy Vegetables, Fruits, Eggs, Chicken, Turkey.

Although the Olive Flame Weightloss Program does not necessarily come with a physical exercise component, and indeed is quite effective without one, some degree of exercise is always more beneficial than none at all. Latest research by Scientists reveals that if you're overweight or obese, rather than doing prolonged moderate exercise such as 30 to 90 minutes of moderate activity on an average of 4 days each week, it is much more beneficial to do intense exercise for a brief period of time frequently.

For example although a 30minute jog does have its benefits, a sudden 3-5 minute intensive sprint within the moderate 30 minute jog will work wonders for you. The same applies to other forms of exercise; brief but intense is more beneficial than sustained but moderate. Put simply, 5 minutes of intensive exercise aids weight loss much better than 30 minutes of moderate exercise. 'Cardio Training', such as cycling, running, stepping, aerobics and walking, is instrumental in weightloss. Additionally it may improve your energy levels and mood, lowering your risk for developing chronic diseases of lifestyle. Also, in addition to 'Cardio training' and right eating, Fitness-Trainers tell us that long-term weight management can be aided by one or two sessions of "Weight training" per week. Key words that come to mind to describe 'Weight training' are dumbbells, therabands, and other specialized gym equipment. Weight training assists in increasing your lean muscle mass. In medical language, it is said that muscles atrophy (wear out) if not used. To kick-start fatloss, "Cardio training" is by far more beneficial. However it is the weight training that helps you sustain the weight loss in the long term. Please note that increasing lean muscle mass also aids weightloss tremendously because lean muscle requires a lot of energy to be maintained, which implies the burning of fat.

Food Diary

Please research ideas of how to draft your own Food Diary, which diary you must use to track your eating patterns during the program. This will help you trace areas where you may not be eating correctly or overeating in the event that your weightloss stalls. If you like you may search the internet for templates of Food Diaries that you may like, via search engines like *google.com.* Some good templates for a Food Diary may be found at *sheknows.com* Diet & Fitness Experts, as well as *theofficediet.com* under Food Diary Templates.

Dietary Guidelines by Blood Types O, A, B, & AO

People of different Blood Types respond differently to different foods. Certain foods tend to promote optimal health much more in people of certain blood groups than people of other blood groups.

Similarly, certain foods trigger diseases or hypersensitivities in people of particular blood groups whilst actually promoting optimal health in people of other blood groups. This phenomenon is based mainly on the existence of particular proteins in food that are called Lectins. Different Lectins in different foods trigger different responses in people of different blood types.

There are 4 Blood Groups in the human family, namely: Type O, Type A, Type B, and Type AB. Please find below tables that give generalized as well as detailed guidelines on the best food choices for people of different blood types to assist you not only with weightloss but the facilitation of optimal health in general by eating foods that are compatible with your blood type. The Tables are courtesy of Michael Lam, MD, MPH, of the Blood Type Diet fame. (www.DrLam.com)

Blood Type Dietary Guidelines - Type O
Courtesy of Michael Lam, MD, MPH
http://www.DrLam.com

Characteristics of Type O - Best on High Protein Diet

1. Thrive on intense physical exercise and animal proteins
2. Do not do well with dairy and grain products
3. Hardy digestive tract
4. The leading factor in weight gain for Type Os is the gluten found in wheat germ and whole wheat products.
5. Type Os have a tendency to have low levels of thyroid hormone and unstable thyroid functions, which cause metabolic problems and weight gain.
6. Type Os have high stomach-acid content, and can digest meat easily.

	Comments	Most Beneficial	Food allowed	Food not allowed
Protein	The more stressful your job or demanding your exercise program, the higher the grade of protein you should eat.	Beef, Lam, Mutton, Veal, Venison.		
	Type Os can efficiently digest and metabolize meats.		Any meat except for those listed as not allowed	Bacon, Ham, Goose, Pork
	Cold-water fish are excellent for Type Os. Many sea foods are also excellent sources of iodine, which regulates the thyroid function.	Cod, herring, Mackerel	Any fish or seafood except for those listed as not allowed	Barracuda, Pickled herring, Catfish, Smoked salmon, Caviar, Octopus, Conch
Dairy	Type Os need to severely restrict the use of dairy products and eggs		Butter, Farmer, Feta, Mozzarella, Goat cheese, Soy Milk	All other dairy products and yogurts
Fat	Type Os respond well to oils	Olive Oil, Flaxseed oil	Canola oil, Sesame Oil	Corn oil, Peanut oil, Cottonseed oil, Safflower oil

	These vegetables irritate the digestive tract and the high mold count can aggravate Type O hypersensitivi ty problems.			Alfalfa sprouts, shiitake mushrooms, fermented olives
	These vegetables can cause arthritic conditions in Type Os			Nightshades: eggplant, potatoes
	These foods affect the production of insulin, often lead to obesity and diabetes for the Type Os.			Corn
	This fruit agglutinate s all blood types but Type Os.		Tomatoes	
		Artichoke, Chicory, Dandelion, Garlic, Horseradish, Kale, Leek, Okra, Onions, Parsley, Parsnips, Red Peppers, Sweet potatoes, Pumpkin, Seaweed, Turnips	All kinds except tho se listed as not allowed	Avocado
Fruits	Dark red, blue and purple fruits tend to cause an alkaline reaction the digestive tract, and therefore balance the high acidity of the Type Os digestive tract to reduce ulcers and irritations of the stomach lining.	Plums, Prunes, Figs		
	These fruits contain high mold counts which can aggravate Type Os hypersensitivity problems (allergies)			Melons, Cantaloupe, Honeydew

	These fruits are high in acid content which may irritate the acidic stomach of Type Os		Grapefruit, most berries	Oranges, tangerines and strawberries, blackberries, Rhubarb
	Fruits are not only an important source of fiber, minerals and vitamins, but they can be an excellent alternative to bread and pasta for Type Os		All kinds except those listed as not allowed	
	Type Os are extremely sensitive to this fruit.			Coconut and Coconut-containing products
Spices	Rich source of Iodine to regulate the thyroid gland	Kelp-based seasonings, Iodized salt		
	Soothing to the digestive tracts of Type Os	Parsley, Curry, Cayenne pepper		
	Irritants to the Type O stomach			White and black pepper, vinegar, capers, cinnamon, Cornstarch, Corn syrup, Nutmeg, Vanilla
Condiments			Chocolate, Honey, cocoa	Ketchup, pickles, mayonnaise, relish
Beverages		Seltzer water, Club Soda and Tea	Wine	Beer, Coffee, Distilled liquor, Black Tea

Blood Type Dietary Guidelines - Type A
Courtesy of Michael Lam, MD, MPH
www.DrLam.com

	Comments	Most Beneficial	Food allowed	Food not allowed
Characteristics of Type A - Best on Vegetarian Diet				
1) Type As are predisposed to Heart Disease, Diabetes, and Cancer and must get their food in as pure a state as possible; fresh, pure and organic. 2) Type As that follow this eating plan will lose weight rather rapidly and potentially short-circuit the development of life-threatening diseases. 3) Good protein sources for Type As are nuts, seeds, vegetable proteins, e.g. in beans and legumes. 4) Dairy foods are poorly digested by Type As. Tofu should be a staple.				
Meats and Poultry	Type As should eliminate all meats from their diet.		Chicken, Cornish hens, Turkey	Beef, Pork, Lamb, Veal, Venison, Duck, Goose
Seafood		Carp, Cod, Grouper, Mackerel, Monkfish, Pickerel, Red snapper, Rainbow trout, Salmon, Sardine, Sea trout, Silver perch, Snail, Whitefish, Yellow Perch	All kinds except those listed as not allowed	Anchovy, Barracuda, Beluga, Bluefish, Bluegill bass, Catfish, Caviar, Clam, Conch, Crab, Crayfish, Eel, Flounder, Frog, Gray sole, Haddock, Hake, Halibut, Herring, Lobster, Lox, Mussels, Octopus, Oysters, Scallop, Shad, Shrimp, Sold, Squid, Striped bass, Tilefish. Turtle
Dairy	Most dairy products are not digestible for Type As		Yogurt, Mozzarella, Feta, Goat cheese, Goat milk, Kefir, Ricotta, String cheese	All other cheeses and milk
Fats		Flaxseed oil, Olive oil	Canola Oil, Cod liver oil	Oil of corn, cottonseed, peanut, safflower and sesame
Nuts		Peanuts, Pumpkin Seeds	All kinds except those listed as not allowed	Brazil nuts, cashews, Pistachios

31

	Type As thrive on the vegetable proteins found in beans and legumes	Beans (Aduke, Azuki, Black, Green, Pinto, Red soy), Lentils and Black-eyed peas	All kinds except those listed as not allowed	
Grains	Type As generally do well on cereals and grains. Select the more concentrated whole grains instead of instant and processed cereals.	Amaranth, Buckwheat		Cream of wheat, Familia, Farina, Granola, Grape nuts, Wheat germ, Seven grain, Shredded wheat, Wheat bran, Durum wheat
Bread & Noodles	Type As have a wonderful selection and choices in grains and pastas	Bread (Essene, Ezekiel, Soya flour, Sprouted wheat), Rice cakes, Flour (Oat, Rice, Rye), Soba Noodles, Pasta (Artichoke)	All kinds except those listed as not allowed	English muffins, Bread (High-protein whole wheat, Multi-grain), Matzos, pumpernickel, Wheat bran muffins, Flour (white, whole wheat), Pasta (Semolina, spinach)
Vegetables	Type As are very sensitive to these vegetables. They have a strong deleterious effect on the Type A digestive tract.			Peppers, olives, Potatoes, Sweet potatoes, Yams, All kinds of cabbage, Tomatoes, Lima beans, Eggplant, Mushroom
	These vegetables enhance the immune system of Type As	Garlic, Onions, Broccoli, carrots, collard greens, kale, pumpkin, spinach		
	Vegetables are vital to the Type A diet, providing minerals, enzymes and Antioxidants. Eat vegetables in as natural a state as possible (raw or steamed) to preserve	Artichoke, Chicory, Greens (Dandelion, Swiss Chard), Horseradish, Leek, Romaine, Okra, Parsley, Alfalfa Sprouts, Tempeh, Tofu, Turnip	All kinds except those listed as not allowed	

Fruits	Most fruits are allowed for Type As, although try to emphasize more alkaline fruits can help to balance the grains that are acid forming in Type As muscle tissues	Berries (blackberries, blueberries, boysenberries, cranberries), plums, Prunes, Figs	All kinds except those listed as not allowed	
	High mold counts of these fruits make it hard for Type As to digest			Melons, cantaloupe, honeydew
	Type As don't do well on these fruits			Mangoes, papaya, Bananas, Coconuts
	These fruits are stomach irritant for Type As, and they also interfere with the absorption of minerals.			Orange, Rhubarb, Tangerines
	The digestive enzyme in this fruit is an excellent digestive aid for Type As	Pineapples, Cherries, Apricots		
	These fruits exhibit alkaline tendencies after digestion which has a positive effects on the Type A stomach	Grapefruit, Lemon		
Spices	The right combination of spices can be powerful immune-system boosters for Type As	Tamari, Miso, Soy-sauce, Garlic, Ginger		
	Good source of iron, a mineral that is lacking in the Type A Diet	Blackstrap molasses		
	Avoid these because the acids tend to cause stomach lining irritation			Vinegar, Pepper (black, cayenne, white), Capers, Plain Gelatin, Wintergreen
Condiments	These products should be avoided because Type			Ketchup, Mayonnaise,

Spices	The right combination of spices can be powerful immune-system boosters for Type As	Tamari, Miso, Soy-sauce, Garlic, Ginger	
	Good source of iron, a mineral that is lacking in the Type A Diet	Blackstrap molasses	
	Avoid these because the acids tend to cause stomach lining irritation		Vinegar, Pepper (black, cayenne, white), Capers, Plain Gelatin, Wintergreen
Condiments	These products should be avoided because Type As have low levels of stomach acid		Ketchup, Mayonnaise, Pickles, Relish, Worcestershire sauce
Beverages	These beverages help to improve the immune systems for Type As	Hawthorn, Aloe, Alfalfa, Burdock, Echinacea, Green tea, Red wine (1 glass / day)	
	These beverages help Type As to increase their stomach-acid secretions	Ginger, Slippery elm, Coffee (1 cup / day)	
	These don't suit the digestive system of Type As, nor do they support the immune system		Beer, Distilled liquor, Seltzer water, Soda, Black Tea

Blood Type Dietary Guidelines - Type B Courtesy of Michael Lam, MD, MPH http://www.DrLam.com

Characteristics of Type B - Best on Balanced Omnivores Diet
1) Type Bs are usually able to resist many of the most severe diseases common to modern life, such as heart disease and cancer but are more prone to immune-system disorders such as multiple sclerosis, lupus, and chronic fatigue syndrome.
2) For Type Bs, the biggest factors in weight gain are corn, buckwheat, lentils, peanuts and sesame seeds.
3) It is important to leave off chicken for Type Bs. Chicken contains a Blood Type B agglutinating lectin in its muscle tissue, which attack the bloodstream and potentially lead to strokes and immune disorders. Type Bs thrive on deep-ocean fish, but should avoid all shellfish. The shellfish contain lectins that are disruptive to the Type B system.
4) Type B is the only blood type that can fully enjoy a variety of dairy foods.
5) Wheat is not tolerated well by most Type Bs.
6) Eliminate tomatoes completely from Type B diet. They have lectins that irritate the stomach lining.

	Comments	Most Beneficial	Food allowed	Food not allowed
Meat and Poultry	These meats contain a Type B blood agglutinating lectin (proteins in food that can cause health problems depending on one's blood type).			Chicken, Cornish hens, Duck, Goose, Partridge, Quail, Pork
	These meats help to boost the immune system	lamb, mutton, Venison, Rabbit		
	Give up chicken, but use these meats instead		Beef, Pheasant, Turkey, Veal	
Seafood	Deep-ocean fish and white fish are great for Type Bs	Cod, Salmon, Flounder, Halibut, Sole. Trout	All kinds except those listed as not allowed	
	These seafoods are poorly digested by Type Bs. They are disruptive to the Type B system.			All Shellfish (crab, shrimp, lobster, mussels, oysters, crayfish, clam, etc), Anchovy, Barracuda, Beluga. Eel. Frog, Lox.

		Bananas, Cranberries, Grapes, Papaya, Plums	All kinds except those listed as not allowed	
Spices	Sweet herbs tend to be stomach irritants to the Type Bs			Barley malt sweeteners, corn syrup, Cornstarch, Cinnamon
	Type B do best with warming herbs	Ginger, horseradish, curry, cayenne pepper	All kinds except those listed as not allowed	
	Avoid these spices also			Allspice, Almond extract, Gelatin, Pepper (black and white)
Condiments				Ketchup
Beverages	Generally Type Bs don't reap overwhelming benefits from most herbal teas.	Ginger, Peppermint, Raspberry leaf, Rose hips, Sage, Green Teas		Aloe, Coltsfoot, Corn silk, Fenugreek, Gentian, Goldenseal, Hops, Linden, Mullein, Red clover, Rhubarb, Senna, Shepherd's purse, Skullcap
	This is highly recommended for Type Bs because it seems to have a positive effect on the nervous system.	Ginseng		
	This has antiviral properties.	Licorice		Distilled liquor, Seltzer water, Soda

Blood Type Dietary Guidelines - Type AB
Courtesy of Michael Lam, MD, MPH
www.DrLam.com

Characteristics of Type AB - Best on Mixed Diet in moderation				
1)				
	Comments	Most Beneficial	Food allowed	Food not allowed
Meat and Poultry	Type AB do not produce enough stomach acid to effectively digest too much animal protein. So the key is portion size and frequency.	Lamb, mutton, rabbit, turkey	All kinds except those listed as not allowed	Beef, Chicken, Cornish Hens, Duck, Goose, Pork, Partridge, Veal, Venison, Quail
	Cured meats can cause stomach cancer Type ABs with low levels of stomach acid			
Seafood	If you have family history of breast cancer, introduce snails (Helix pomatia) into your diet	Tuna, Cod, Grouper, Hake, Mackerel, Mahimahi, Monkfish, Ocean Perch, Pike, Porgy, Trout, Red Snapper, Sailfish, Pickerel, Sardine, Shad, Snail, Sturgeon	All kinds except those listed as not allowed	All Shellfish (crab, shrimp, lobster, mussels, oysters, crayfish, clam, etc), Anchovy, Barracuda, Beluga, Bluegill Bass, Flounder, Haddock, Halibut, Herring, Eel, Frog, Lox, Octopus, Sea bass, Striped bass, Turtle, Yellowtail
Dairy	Cultured and soured products are easily digested for Type ABs	Yogurt, Kefir, Non-fat sour cream, egg, Mozzarella, Goat cheese and milk, Ricotta	All kinds except those listed as not allowed	American Cheese, Blue cheese, Brie, Buttermilk, Camembert, Ice cream, Parmesan, Provolone, Sherbet, Whole Milk
Fats	Use sparingly	Olive		Oil (Corn, Cottonseed, Safflower, Sesame, Sunflower)

Fats	Use sparingly	Olive		Oil (Corn, Cottonseed, Safflower, Sesame, Sunflower)
Nuts	Powerful immune booster for Type A and Type AB	Peanut, Walnuts		
	Type ABs tend to suffer from gallbladder problems, so nut butters are preferable to whole nuts. Also eat small amounts with caution.		All kinds except those listed as not allowed	Filberts, Poppy seeds, Pumpkin seeds, Sesame seeds, Sunflower seeds
Beans	These beans are important cancer-fighting food for Type AB. They are known to contain cancer-fighting antioxidants.	Lentils		
	These beans slow insulin production in Type AB.			Kidney beans, Lima Beans
		Beans (navy, pinto, red, soy)	All kinds except those listed as not allowed	Beans (Aduke, Azuki, Black, Fava, Garbanzo) Black-eyed Peas
Grains	The inner kernel of the wheat grain is highly acid forming for Type AB. Wheat is not advised if Type AB is trying to lose weight. The inner kernel of wheat grain is alkaline in Type Os and Bs, it becomes acidic in Type As and AB.	Millet, Oat bran, Oatmeal, Rice Bran, Puffed rice, Rye, Spelt and sprouted wheat and any products such as flour, bread and noodles made with these grain products	All kinds except those listed as not allowed	Buckwheat, Corn (any products such as flour, bread and noodles made with these), Kamut, Kasha, soba noodles, Artichoke pasta
	Type AB benefits from a diet rich in rice rather than pasta	All kinds of Rice and any products such as flour, bread and		

Vegetables	Fresh vegetables are an important source of phytochemicals which have a tonic effect in cancer and heart disease prevention. These diseases afflict Type AB more often as a result of weaker immune system.	Broccoli, Beets, Cauliflower, Celery, Green Leafy Veges, Cucumber, Eggplant, Garlic, Maitake Mushroom, Parsley, Parsnips, Sweet potatoes, Alfalfa Sprouts, Tempeh, Tofu, All types of Yams	All kinds except those listed as not allowed	Artichoke, Avocado, All types of Corns, Lima Beans, Black Olives, All kind of Bell Peppers, Radishes, Mung Bean Sprouts, Radish Sprouts
Fruits	Emphasize the more alkaline fruits to balance the grains that are acid forming in Type AB muscle tissues	All kinds of Grapes and Plums, Berries (cranberries, Gooseberries, Loganberries), Cherries		
	Tropical fruits doesn't agree with Type AB. But pineapple is an excellent digestive aid for Type AB.	Pineapples		Mangoes, Guava, Coconuts, Bananas
	Oranges are stomach irritant for Type AB, they also interfere with the absorption of important minerals. But Grapefruit exhibit alkaline tendencies after digestion. And lemons aid digestion and clearing mucus from the system.	Grapefruits, Lemons		Oranges
	Vitamin C-rich fruits help prevent stomach cancer because of the antioxidant properties of vitamin cup	Kiwi	All kinds except those listed as not allowed	
Spices	Sea salt and kelp should be used in place of salt. Kelp has immensely	Kelp, Miso, Curry	All kinds except those	Allspice, Almond extract, Anise, Barley

39

Spices	Sea salt and kelp should be used in place of salt. Kelp has immensely positive heart and immune system benefits	Kelp, Miso, Curry	All kinds except those listed as not allowed	Allspice, Almond extract, Anise, Barley Malt, Capers, Cornstarch, corn syrup, Gelatin, Tapioca
	The ingredients are acidic			Vinegar, Pepper (white, black, cavenne, red flakes)
	This is a potent tonic and natural antibiotic for Type AB.	Garlic, Horseradish, Parsley		
Beverages	Type AB employed these herbal teas to rev up the immune system.	Alfalfa, burdock, Chamomile, Echinacea, Green tea		
	These herbal teas and beverages build protections against cardiovascular disease and cancer.	Hawthorn, Licorice, Red wine (1 glass/day)		
	These herbal teas aid in absorption of iron and prevent anemia	Dandelion, Burdock root, Strawberry leaf		
	Coffee increase stomach acid and has the same enzymes found in soy.	Coffee or Decaf Coffee (1 cup / day) and alternate day use green tea		Distilled Liquor, Sodas, Black Tea

About the Author

Humphrey Zinyuke (BSc Nutrition) is a free-lance author and qualified Nutritionist. He is also a keen student of demography and popular-culture.

A drummer in a band, Humphrey enjoys The Discovery Channel, English Premiership League Football, and the music of Six-Pence-None-The Richer, if he's not busy socializing on Twitter, Facebook, or trying to figure out how Pinterest works.

Other Titles by this Author:

THE EROS MYSTIQUE: Investigating the New Sexual World Order
You can find it on Facebook on the page: THE EROS MYSTIQUE

Connect with Humphrey Online:

Facebook: http://www.facebook.com/OliveFlameWeightLossProgram
                http://www.facebook.com/zinyuke
Twitter: @OliveFlameDiet/ #OliveFlameDiet
Email: oliveflamenutrition@gmail.com